10-Day
Celery Juice
Cleanse

An Hachette Company
www.hachette.co.uk

First published in Great Britain in 2019 by Aster,
an imprint of Octopus Publishing Group Ltd
Carmelite House
50 Victoria Embankment
London EC4Y 0DZ
www.octopusbooks.co.uk

First published in paperback 2020

Distributed in the US by
Hachette Book Group
1290 Avenue of the Americas
4th and 5th Floors
New York, NY 10104

Distributed in Canada by
Canadian Manda Group
664 Anette Street., Toronto,
Ontario, Canada M6S 2CB

ISBN: 978-1-78325-365-4

Consultant Publisher: Kate Adams
Copy Editor: Jane Birch
Designer: Jeremy Tilston
Cover image: Sunstock/iStock

10-Day Celery Juice Cleanse

The fresh start plan to supercharge your health

HANNAH EBELTHITE & KATE ADAMS

CONTENTS

WHY IS EVERYONE TALKING ABOUT CELERY JUICE?

If you have even a passing interest in health and wellbeing, you can't fail to have noticed the growing interest a certain crunchy, green salad vegetable. Especially when enjoyed in liquid form. Celery juice is being hailed as the latest superfood, the must-drink of the moment. Like so many modern trends, the word has spread via social media, with Instagram in particular being a vehicle for fans to share their snaps of vibrant green juice alongside rave reports of its effects. At the time of writing, the hashtag #celeryjuice had been used over 185,000 times. Recent reports have even suggested that the craze is driving up the price of celery in supermarkets in parts of North America.

Celery is an obvious health food by virtue of it being a vegetable – we all know greens are good for us. But its current spell in the spotlight is largely down to Anthony Williams, aka the 'Medical Medium', who desribes himself as the 'originator of the celery juice movement'. An author and self-styled health expert (he's open about having no medical or scientific qualification), he claims to be able to 'read' people's health. Since the age of four, he's been intuiting messages that celery juice is 'a miracle juice, one of the greatest healing tonics of all time'. With plenty of celebrity fans and legions of online influencers supporting his claims and sharing their own anecdotes of healing and greater health, it's no surprise the word has spread. So, should we all be downing a daily glass of green goodness?

Let's look at the claims being made about celery and its juice, its known nutritional status and the research that supports its health benefits.

Then, after considering its traditional medicinal and culinary uses, you can decide for yourself whether this humble green vegetable deserves a starring role in your daily diet.

CHAPTER 1

WHAT'S THE NUTRITIONAL LOW-DOWN?

Until recently, celery might not have been on your nutrition radar. It's certainly not been at the top of any superfood charts. But that's perhaps unfair because these humble green sticks pack a whole bunch of goodness. We all know how important it is to consume more vegetables and fruit, with five a day a recommended minimum. Munching on just one and a half full-length celery sticks counts as one portion towards your daily quota.

With nutrition and environmental experts worldwide extolling the benefits of a more plant-based diet, we should all be expanding our vegetable repertoire.

Like all veggies, celery is very low in calories, fat and cholesterol. It has a high water and electrolyte content, at least 90 per cent, so it is hydrating, too. It's a low-carbohydrate food but still a decent source of fibre (if that's not removed by juicing), so it supports healthy digestion and may aid weight loss. In fact, celery is one of the very best sources of prebiotic fibre, which is the food which trillions of friendly microbes in our gut need to thrive and multiply. Gut health is one of the most researched and exciting areas of medicine at the moment, with new evidence constantly emerging to suggest that an abundant and diverse microbiome means better overall physical and mental health as well as a reduced risk of a whole host of conditions.

Eating celery provides you with a good range of vitamins, minerals and antioxidants, including vitamins K, A, B6 and C, folate, riboflavin, potassium, manganese, calcium and magnesium. It's a good source of beneficial enzymes and contains compounds that help it act as a diuretic and reduce water retention and bloating. Its phytonutrients also include flavonoids and polyphenols, which have linked the vegetable to better liver, eye, skin and cognitive health.

A zero-waste food, you can enjoy every part of a celery plant – sticks, leaves, seeds, even the root (as in celeriac, a related plant). And it's one of the most versatile vegetables as you can have it raw, in salads and crudités, juiced or blended into smoothies and soups, steamed as a side dish or added to countless cooked dishes such as risottos, sauces, ragùs and stews. Celery seeds can be bought whole, crushed or ground and used as a spice or salt – the distinctive flavour comes from the oily compound, apiol, contained in the vegetable.

If you're trying to lose weight or maintain your healthy weight, raw celery is an excellent addition to your daily diet. Studies have shown foods with a satisfying crunch help you to feel fuller for longer. Munching on some celery sticks can easily become a mindful-eating exercise that really helps you enjoy its flavour and texture as well as appreciate its goodness. As a sustaining and delicious snack, try dipping celery sticks in some nut butter or houmous for an extra hit of protein and healthy fats.

Caution: celery is among a small group of foods that can cause potentially fatal anaphylactic shock in susceptible people (similar to a peanut allergy) If you have food allergies it's worth speaking to your doctor or a dietitian to establish risk.

WHAT ARE THE CLAIMS?

Members of the 'celery juice movement' claim it has profound healing effects that can change the lives of those battling chronic illness. The list of conditions it's been claimed a daily juice can help is lengthy, ranging from chronic fatigue syndrome (CFS/ME) to eczema, fibromyalgia to psoriasis and even cancer. The fact these claims have yet to be substantiated isn't of concern to Williams, who simply says that science hasn't got there yet. His source, he insists, is 'the spirit' who communicates with him. His proof? The thousands of supporters who confirm the positive effects on their own health. 'Celery juice is not easy to make and it doesn't taste very good, so for it to thrive to this degree is testament,' he has said.

The Medical Medium website says celery juice is saving lives as it restores people's health, one symptom at a time. It claims the juice can:

- Heal the gut and relieve digestive disorders
- Balance blood sugar, blood pressure, weight and adrenal function
- Neutralize and flush toxins from the liver and brain
- Provide the brain with electrolyte support to counter disease

- Treat a vast range of chronic and mystery illnesses, including fatigue, brain fog, acne, eczema, addiction, attention deficit hyperactivity disorder (ADHD), thyroid disorders, diabetes, small intestinal bacterial overgrowth (SIBO), eating disorders, autoimmune disorders, Lyme disease and eye problems

As a digestive aid, celery juice is claimed to be a natural laxative, to reduce inflammation in the gut and to increase absorption of other nutrients in your diet. It's said to contain enzymes that raise levels of hydrochloric acid in your stomach to aid digestion and prevent fermentation in the gut and therefore bloating. And those who believe in an alkaline diet say celery juice helps to alkalinize the gut.

Many of the effects Williams puts down to his claim that celery contains substances called cluster salts, an 'undiscovered' subgroup of salt, that kill off pathogens like bacteria and viruses.

Williams' protocol is to drink 16oz (473ml or almost 1 pint) of pure celery juice every morning on an empty stomach, then wait 15 minutes before eating any other food. If you really don't like the taste or find the amount hard to ingest, he concedes that you can add an apple or some cucumber, and start with half the amount. But the goal is to phase out additional ingredients and build up to the full dose of pure celery.

ARE THERE ANY STUDIES INTO THE HEALTH BENEFITS?

The long list of claims made by the Medical Medium and other advocates on social media suggests celery juice is nothing short of a miracle. But what does the science really say?

First, we must acknowledge that facts about dietary discoveries are rarely as simple as headlines might promise. Research into the effects of a single food is notoriously hard to carry out. It's incredibly difficult to analyse how one small element of our diet affects our health as a whole. Why? Well, human cohort studies that rely on accurate self-reporting are notoriously flawed. And, of course, there are many other confounding factors that could skew results, such as the rest of a person's complex diet, their exercise and lifestyle habits or existing health conditions, to name just a few.

As such, many of the scientific studies behind the headlines – for all foods, not just celery – will have been performed in more controlled conditions on animals. Or even using isolated compounds from food in Petri dishes. In other words, we can only guess that the findings can be extrapolated to real people eating real food in varying quantities.

Of course, that's not to say that any findings are nonsense. We can think of them as valuable first steps. Absence of proof is not proof of absence and, as with many nutritional and complementary therapies, thousands of years of anecdotal evidence is what convinces many people that there are real health benefits to be had. But let's look at the existing science for the moment. Here's what research suggests celery may offer us.

HEART HEALTH BENEFITS

Celery contains antioxidants and has been shown in pharmacological studies to demonstrate activity that may help reduce blood pressure and cholesterol levels, lowering heart disease risk – although the blood pressure reduction does seem to come from the seeds rather than the sticks.

A 2013 human study gave 30 volunteers with hypertension celery seed extract (not juice) for six weeks. There was a statistically significant decrease in blood pressure over that time, although this study had no control group and the authors were linked to the supplement used.

Researchers from the University of Chicago Medical Center identified an oil compound in celery that can reduce blood pressure by relaxing the smooth muscles that line blood vessels. The chemical, called 3-n-butylphthalide (3nB), which provides celery's distinctive smell and taste, lowered blood pressure in rats by 12 to 14 per cent and cholesterol by 7 per cent. A further rat study, published in the *Journal of Medicinal Food*, also found celery seed extract to be effective at reducing chronic hypertension.

It appears the 3nB compounds reduce blood pressure by acting as both a diuretic and vasodilator (working in a similar way to prescribed drugs). Because this doesn't change the ratio of sodium to potassium in the blood, as pharmaceutical diuretics do, celery seed extract has the potential to offer the same benefits without dangerous side effects.

Other studies on rats fed a high fat diet have demonstrated reduced blood lipids (cholesterol levels) in those also given liquid celery extract.

ANTI-INFLAMMATORY PROPERTIES

Celery is high in antioxidant flavones and polyphenols, which are known to have an anti-inflammatory effect. They protect the body against free radical damage (oxidative stress) that over time can lead to inflammation. A study published in *Molecular Nutrition & Food Research* concluded that apigenin (a type of flavone in celery) and apigenin-rich diets may help reduce inflammation and restore immune balance. Inflammation is a big factor in many chronic diseases such as cancer, heart disease, arthritis, gout, skin disorders like acne, psoriasis, rosacea, irritable bowel syndrome (IBS) and more.

NEUROGENESIS

The apigenin in celery is also thought to stimulate neurogenesis (growth and development of nerve cells). A 2009 mice study found it improved learning and memory.

PROTECTS LIVER HEALTH

Again, this was a study on rats, but Egyptian researchers found that supplementing a high-cholesterol diet with celery and chicory leaves and barley powder saw improvements in liver enzyme function and lipid levels. Liver enzymes help break down proteins for the body to absorb and detoxify chemicals and alcohol.

REDUCES BLOATING AND BOOSTS DIGESTION

Bloating in this instance means water retention (rather than gas) and this effect comes from the same diuretic properties that also make celery useful for high blood pressure. In terms of digestion, effects may vary. Increasing fibre intake may be useful for some people and not others. Celery is a high FODMAP food (it contains mannitol) – FODMAPs are compounds thought to trigger digestive problems – so may worsen bloating and other digestive issues in those with IBS. On a low FODMAP diet, no more than 10g of whole celery is recommended so a glass of juice would be too much.

FIGHTS INFECTION

Studies confirm the traditional use of celery seeds to boost immunity and fight infection. A 2009 report in the *Journal of Pharmacy and Pharmacology* identified compounds with antimicrobial properties.

By stimulating urine production and removing uric acid, celery may also help protect against urinary tract infections (UTIs).

ULCER AND CANCER PROTECTIVE

A 2010 study published in the *Journal of Pharmaceutical Biology* identifies a type of ethanol extract found in celery that can replenish gastric mucus in the digestive tract, protecting against ulcers. Certain chemical constituents may also help control the level of gastric acid released.

There's also a 2014 study, which found apigenin treatment produced a reduction in the rate of gastritis and gastric cancers in gerbils infected with heliobacter plyori (a bacteria that causes stomach ulcers, inflammation and increases cancer risk).

Celery contains the flavonoid luteolin, which researchers believe may have anti-cancer properties. A study in *Current Cancer Drug Targets* says luteolin may make cancer cells more susceptible to attack by drug treatment.

A 2009 study on rats found the juice of celery leaves may help to reduce the cardiotoxic side effects of a chemotherapy drug.

By adding celery and/or its juice to an otherwise healthy, balanced diet, you could well see some benefits due your increased intake of vitamins, minerals, antioxidants, phytochemicals and even fluids. You might see benefits to your skin, hair, nails, energy levels, or improvements in blood pressure or any inflammatory conditions you suffer from. And it's worth remembering that there are lots of other green vegetables that offer similar or greater benefits, such as broccoli, kale, and wheatgrass.

CHAPTER 2

CELERY AND ITS TRADITIONAL USES

Celery, scientific name *Apium graveolens*, belongs the Apiaceae plant family. Other members include carrots, parsnips, parsley and celeriac. It's native to the Mediterranean and Middle East but now grown in many parts of the world. The type of celery we know today, with its tall, fleshy sticks was only developed in the late 18th century.

Wild celery, however, has been around since ancient times, with records suggesting celery leaves were found in Tutankhamun's tomb in ancient Egypt. The Greeks valued celery as an aphrodisiac, a flavouring and to make wine. It's mentioned in *The Iliad* and *The Odyssey* by Homer – horses ate the wild celery that grew in Troy. The Romans used celery leaves to make wreaths or crowns for those victorious in battles. They also used it to cure hangovers (and this may be why a stick of celery is used in modern-day Bloody Mary cocktails). In ancient China, celery was used for medicinal properties.

For centuries, celery has been an anti-hypertensive agent in folk medicine, used to bring down high blood pressure. The seeds are known for their diuretic and kidney-stimulating action. This may flush out excess uric acid and crystals that could otherwise cause problems like gout, arthritis and kidney stones. By increasing urine output and removing toxins it's thought to be 'cleansing'. Its seeds are thought to relieve pain.

In Traditional Chinese Medicine (TCM), celery is also used to treat high blood pressure, as well as being a general qi (energy) tonic. It's used in medicines to tonify the spleen and stomach, aid digestion, and reduce flatulence and loss of appetite. It's energizing, cools the liver and treats headaches, period pain, menopausal disorders, gout and rheumatism. It purifies the blood, promotes sweating and easing colds, flu and fevers. By promoting urination, it cleanses the kidney and bladder and relieves heat in the body. It stops bleeding, thereby helping heavy periods, wounds or ulcers.

In Ayurvedic medicine, celery seeds are valued for their ability to help the body regulate itself. They're used to treat various ailments including flu, colds and arthritis. They are thought to be generally useful for digestive disorders, relieving bloating and flatulence and promoting healthy bowel movements.

The seeds also have a traditional use in regulating menstrual flow and cycles, and relieving cramps and premenstrual syndrome (PMS) – this may be thanks to the plant chemical apiol and its effects on the endocrine system.

Celery and its seeds have calming and sedative properties because of the phytochemical limonene, so it could be a good food and medicine in times of stress.

CHAPTER 3

GROWING, BUYING, STORING AND JUICING CELERY

Celery is a long-season crop that can be rather a challenge for gardeners. It needs to be sown indoors then transferred to deep trenches outside (as you would grow leeks). It likes cool, moist climates and needs constant watering. But with a little time and effort, you could have a satisfying yield from your home veggie patch or allotment.

If you don't have the ability or inclination to grow your own, celery is widely available year-round from greengrocers and in the salad aisle in supermarkets. Try to buy locally produced celery where you can to reduce unnecessary carbon emissions through air and road miles.

Celery is a heavily sprayed crop with multiple pesticides so stick to organic where possible or wash well with diluted apple cider vinegar before using.

Healthy, fresh celery should have brightly coloured leaves and firm, not bendy, sticks. It can be bought as a whole head or in pre-trimmed sticks. It will store well in the drawer of your refrigerator (it doesn't freeze well) and, while its nutrient content will decrease with time, it can still be used when it starts to go limp. To prepare celery, cut off and discard the base, save the leaves (good in stir-fries, soups and risottos), rinse any soil off the sticks and use as desired.

Thanks to the celery juice trend sweeping the globe, manufacturers are getting in on the act, too. You'll find celery-based juices in health-food stores, delis and supermarkets – even celery-flavoured sodas and mixers. Just beware that any nutritional benefit will be reduced by processing, pasteurizing and storage. By all means try them if you enjoy the flavour, but for health gains, make your own.

Remember that if you're consuming three times more fruit and veg than you normally do, you'll also be ingesting three times as many pesticides, so wash everything thoroughly and choose organic where possible.

JUICING AND BLENDING

Of course, there are countless ways to enjoy whole celery, raw and in cooking. But if the celery juice trend has piqued your interest, you'll be keen to give this green elixir a go. Juicing has become hugely popular in recent years, especially as the equipment needed to do it becomes more advanced, available and affordable. In essence, juicing means extracting the liquid from fruit and vegetables, while removing the fibrous pulp. You're left with a nutrient-packed power drink that's tasty, hydrating, easy on the digestive system and quickly absorbed. In one glass you're getting the concentrated vitamin, mineral and antioxidant content of perhaps five or ten portions of fruit and veg, which you couldn't possibly manage in one sitting if you were to eat it all. (Juicing a whole head of celery, for example, will yield an easy-to-drink glass of between 300 and 500ml/10–18fl oz, whereas crunching your way through the same amount of the vegetable would take quite a while and might give you quite the tummy ache!).

JUICERS

There are two types of juicer (if you don't count the traditional hand reamer you might use to squeeze juice from an orange or lemon): centrifugal juicers use a sharp blade that separates juice from pulp; masticating or slow juicers use an auger to squeeze out the juice. Both require some preparation of the fruit and veg and, depending on its design, it can be a pain to clean out the juicer afterwards.

Masticating juicers, also called 'slow juicers', do extract more nutrients than centrifugal juicers and are particularly suited to juicing celery. They tend to have smaller mesh parts, so save on the washing up.

JUICE CLEANSES OR FASTS

Some fans of juicing advocate juice cleanses or fasts – whole days or even weeks of drinking only juices, to rest the digestive system, cleanse the body of toxins and maximize your vitamin and mineral intake. Others simply believe in a daily or occasional juice to pack in some extra antioxidants from a large amount of fruit and veg they'd be otherwise unable to consume on that day.

Critics of juicing, however, point out that by extracting the pulp, you're not really benefitting from the whole fruit or vegetable. Many nutrients are contained in the peel, seeds or pulp – not least the plant fibre. When there's no fibre present, we absorb not just the good stuff but also the fructose (fruit sugars) in juice much more quickly – because liquids pass through the stomach to the intestine faster than solids.

Vegetable juices tend to contain more nutrients and they naturally have less fructose. However, they're still lacking fibre. This is important not just for keeping our blood sugar levels stable but for helping us feel fuller for longer and for feeding those gut microbes. It's recommended that adults consume 30g (1oz) of fibre each day. Diets high in fibre are linked to a lower risk of coronary heart disease, stroke, high blood pressure and diabetes. So adding celery juice to your daily diet isn't a straight swap for eating whole vegetables – the ideal combination is to have both!

We have included a 3-day juice cleanse in the next chapter if you feel like your digestion is in need of a good rest. Or you can go straight to the 7-day Juice and Soup Cleanse, which is full of healthy juices, smoothies and soups to kickstart your healthy diet.

GREEN SMOOTHIES

If you love juices but want the fibre benefits, too, you can also try using a blender. You add chopped, whole fruit or vegetables into the jug (minus peel or seeds that you wouldn't normally eat) and blend it to a liquid. Any pulp remains in the drink but is puréed. Blending is well suited to soft fruit and vegetables like berries, bananas, avocados and leafy green veg – although you'll probably still need to add water to make a thinner consistency. But it doesn't work so well for fibrous fruit and veg like citrus fruit, apples, root veg or stringy celery.

A couple of solutions: first, if the food has a high water content, like citrus or celery, you can use what's often called a nut milk bag (like a muslin) to strain the blended liquid and remove any pulp that's not nice to drink. With this option, however, we're back to the issue of having removed most of the fibre, if not quite as much as in juicing. Perhaps the best solution, then, is to use a more advanced 'nutrient extractor blender' (such as the Nutribullet). These are powerful blenders that can break down fruit, vegetables, pulses, even nuts, seeds and some grains. Because the juice or smoothie they produce contains more fibre, the drink is more slowly absorbed and blood sugar less elevated.

In short? If making your own healthy drinks, stick to low-sugar vegetables, only adding a little fruit to taste if needed (such as some apple or lemon juice to help your taste buds adjust to celery). And make sure the rest of your diet contains a healthy mix of fibre, protein and fats.

Think of a juice or smoothie as a healthy addition to your diet rather than a meal replacement – the Medical Medium advises drinking your celery juice before breakfast like a medicine, not instead of breakfast. Ideally, don't replace more than one meal a day with a drink, unless you're doing a short juice cleanse.

SO, WHAT'S IT REALLY LIKE TO DRINK CELERY JUICE EVERY DAY?

A quick scroll through Instagram will give you a good insight into the benefits fans of celery juice swear by. Hollywood A-listers and influencers are keen to share their experiences and encourage us all to join in (Gwyneth Paltrow, Elle Macpherson, Sylvester Stallone, Robert De Niro, Novak Djokovic, Miranda Kerr, Pharrell Williams and Calvin Harris have all shared posts). But what can you really expect if you commit?

'I was intrigued to try adding celery juice to my diet first thing in the morning to see whether I would feel any different. I don't have a bad diet generally, but my energy levels have been a bit low and I do suffer from 'brain fog'. After just a couple of days I felt more clear-headed and my digestion feels lighter and not sluggish at all. I also enjoy the ritual of juicing a whole head of celery first thing – it's like a meditation! I have hot water and lemon before the celery juice to ease into it, and I'm lucky that I like the taste of celery.' – Kate

'I've been drinking celery juice for a month now, every morning. I have it after hot lemon and apple cider vinegar. It tasts bitter, I sometimes add cucumber or apple, but honestly I've gotten used to it and actually crave it now. I've noticed less bloating, better digestion, more energy, no stomach cramps, regular and healthier stools. It's definitely kickstarted my healing process from Addison's disease and a leaky gut.' – Fiona

'I started juicing a whole head of celery (organic as I know they're high in pesticides) and drinking it first thing before food. I only have an old juicer someone gave me but it works fine – the only effort is cleaning the blade. I find it really refreshing and I like the taste of celery so that wasn't an issue for me. I found out after just two weeks my eczema had really improved. It didn't clear up 100 per cent so now I'm experimenting and adding other ingredients like apple cider vinegar and spirulina.' – Shona

'I'm a nutritionist and I make a green juice every morning for myself and my clients. I like to start my day with alkalising elements. My favourite combination is two bunches of celery, one bunch of flat-leaf parsley, one or two cucumbers, one or two green apples (for sweetness) and one peeled lime. I use a Hurom masticating juicer as I find the juice lasts longer with this cold-press, slow type.' – Aine

'I definitely feel the health benefits when I drink celery juice. It just feels good for you, it's a nice self-care ritual to start your day. The bright green juice looks bursting with nutrients and I swear wakes me up. After a couple of weeks my skin glows and it seems to nix any breakouts. The only difficulty I have is being organised. I work long hours and don't always remember to stock up on celery. Plus you need to allow time in the morning to wash and prep your celery, juice it, drink it, clean the juicer and then wait half an hour before breakfast. If I'm in a rush, that doesn't always happen!' – Heather

CHAPTER 4

10-DAY CLEANSE

In the following chapters you will find a specially curated 10-day cleanse, the first 3-days are constituted of a juice-based cleanse, followed by a 7-day soup and juice cleanse. You can also jump straight to the soup and juice cleanse if you don't fancy three straight days of juice. The purpose of a cleanse is to give your digestion a rest and reset. It can also be helpful for getting rid of any excess water retention and can be an excellent start to a longer healthy-eating weight loss plan as it shifts your mindset as well as pounds.

Drinking three to five juices per day equates to around 600 to 1000 calories, so following a juice cleanse for several days will help most people to create a calorie deficit and lose one to two kilograms. This sort of diet is not intended for the long term but is designed to reset poor dietary habits and kickstart a new, healthier way of eating. You'll become more in tune with your hunger, aware of how often you were snacking previously – and how unnecessary it was. Your taste buds will become more sensitive, your sweet tooth curbed and you'll probably find that, by the end of the cleanse, processedand sugary foods taste quite unnatural and unpleasant.

Try the following cleanse to give your digestive system a rest, get accustomed to the taste and benefits of celery juice, and set you on a path to new, healthier habits...

Here are some of the benefits you could enjoy:
1. Lose weight
2. Feel less bloated
3. Regular bowel movements
4. Improved sleep
5. Feel more clearheaded

Signs that you might benefit from a cleanse include:

- Low energy
- You feel tired, especially just after eating
- Irregular bowel movements
- Brain fog
- Cravings for foods you know aren't good for you
- You feel bloated

A cleanse is a way to help your body come back into balance by supporting it with simple eating and living for a few days. It is also the perfect time to slow down, clear your diary and rest. In today's busy world, it is easy to feel as though you are running on empty, so a cleanse is a great way of topping up your energy reserves.

WHAT'S IN THE CLEANSE?

As mentioned earlier, vegetable juices are preferred to fruit juices when cleansing as they don't contain so many fruit sugars. The idea of

juicing your vegetables is to make them easy
to digest. There are also a couple of key spices
included in the cleanse which are also supportive
to digestion – ginger and turmeric – plus an
optional oil and juice. Do buy local, organic
ingredients where possible as these are grown
without the levels of pesticides used to grow
non-organic produce.

TURMERIC – THE ANTI-INFLAMMATORY POWERHOUSE

Turmeric is one of nature's most powerful ancient healers and has been used medicinally for over 4,500 years. Modern research into the benefits of turmeric has focused on curcumin, its main active ingredient. This has been shown to have anti-inflammatory effects and it is also an antioxidant. Inflammation has been linked to heart disease, diabetes, Alzheimer's, stroke, arthritis and cancer. Studies also show the potential anti-cancer benefits of turmeric, both as part of a preventative lifestyle and for cancer patients undergoing treatment.

Ginger – gentle fire for the digestion
Ginger is closely related to turmeric and also has anti-inflammatory properties. It is an excellent ingredient for adding to juices (or soups) as it has been shown to help improve the efficiency of digestion in the body. In Chinese medicine and Ayurveda, ginger is described as 'warming', so it helps with the digestive 'fire'.

CBD oil

Another fast-growing trend in health-food stores is kemp-derived CBD (Cannabidiol) oil. CBD is one of the non-psychoactive compounds in cannabis, so it doesn't produce an effect on the mind, and is extracted and diluted in a carrier oil (usually hemp). The main health benefit associated with CBD is in the treatment of pain. Studies are now linking it to potentially helping with the treatment of neurological disorders, reducing anxiety and helping with some of the side effects of chemotherapy treatment. It can easily be added in small quantities to juices.

Aloe vera juice

Aloe vera juice is considered to be anti-inflammatory and therefore may be healing for the digestive tract and may provide some relief for joint pain. You might wish to add a capful (check the directions on the container) to your juices once a day.

WHAT YOU'LL NEED FOR PHASE ONE, THE 3-DAY JUICE CLEANSE

VEG

- Beetroot
- Carrot
- Celery
- Cucumber
- Kale
- Spinach

FRUIT

- Apple
- Lemon juice
- Pineapple

NUTS

- Almonds
- Almond milk

THE JUICES
Celery
- 1 or 1½ head of celery

CELERY+
Celery, apple, lemon
- ½ head celery
- 1 or 2 apples
- Squeeze of lemon juice

COOL DOWN
Celery, apple, cucumber
- 3 sticks celery
- 2 apples
- 1 cucumber

FIRE UP
Apple, carrot, ginger, turmeric, lemon

- 2 apples
- 2 large carrots
- 2.5cm (1in) piece fresh root ginger
- ¼ teaspoon ground turmeric
- Squeeze of lemon juice

ZINGER
Carrot, lemon, ginger

- 4 carrots
- Juice of ¼ lemon
- 2.5cm (1in) piece fresh root ginger

EARTH
Beetroot, ginger, apple

- 2 medium beetroot
- 2 apples
- 2.5cm (1in) piece fresh root ginger

SUNSHINE
Celery, pineapple, cucumber, lime

- 3 celery sticks
- 100g (3½oz) fresh pineapple
- ½ cucumber
- Juice of ½ lime

GREEN
Celery, spinach, kale, cucumber, lime, ginger

- 3 celery sticks
- 50g (1¾oz) spinach
- 50g (1¾oz) kale
- ½ cucumber
- Juice of ½ lime
- 2.5cm (1in) piece fresh root ginger

MAKING YOUR JUICES

Step 1. Rinse all the ingredients well.

Step 2. Peel fruit and veg such as ginger, beetroot and pineapple. There's no need to peel apples or carrots. Roughly chop into 2.5–5cm (1–2in) pieces.

Step 3. Juice following the manufacturer's instructions for your juicer.

OTHER DRINKS

Drink water, ideally at room temperature rather than ice cold, throughout the day. You can flavour your water with lemon or lime, cucumber, rosemary or mint.

If you are feeling brave, then a glass of water each day with a capful of apple cider vinegar will also benefit your digestion.

The best cleansing teas include:

Fennel

Nettle

Dandelion

Green

Fresh mint

And for a warm, healthy boosting drink add a little fresh turmeric root, lemon juice and fresh root ginger to hot water.

It's a good idea to include a nut milk drink each day, if you are able to consume nuts. If not, then add 1 teaspoon of ground flaxseeds to each of your juices.

Cacao Berry Nut Milk

- 250ml (9fl oz) almond milk
- 1 heaped teaspoon cacao powder
- 50g (1¾oz) frozen blueberries

Blitz all the ingredients together.

THE 3-DAY JUICE PLAN

For each day of the juice cleanse, rise on waking and start the day with hot water and a squeeze of lemon juice to warm up your digestion without giving it anything to do.

Make celery juice your first juice of the day and then enjoy six to eight juices of your choice plus one nut milk through the day. Always leave at least 15 minutes between the first celery juice and drinking or eating anything else. Sip room-temperature water and herbal teas throughout the day.

Example day

6.30am: Warm water and lemon juice

7am: Celery Juice

7.30am: Nut milk

10.30am: Sunshine Juice

12.30pm: Green Juice

1pm: Handful of almonds

3pm: Zinger Juice

5pm: Green Juice

7pm: Earth Juice

Extra tips for a cleanse
Write things down

Keeping a journal of how you feel physically, mentally and emotionally is helpful for any change in diet or lifestyle. It's important to find out what feels good for us as individuals as not everyone likes the same ingredients or or is suited to exactly the same ways of eating. It's also a very good way to track whether your sleep, levels of energy and moods begin to balance out.

Skin brushing

Body or skin brushing is something you can do at home every day to help stimulate your circulation. We excrete and eliminate waste products through our skin, just as our liver and kidneys are also organs of elimination. Skin brushing is also thought to support the lymph system that, like the bloodstream, goes all around our bodies, and is a major filtering system for the body as well as helping us to fight infections as part of the immune system.

How to skin brush

Do this on dry skin a couple of minutes before you shower. Use a natural bristled brush, ideally with a long handle so you can reach your back. Don't brush your face or anywhere that feels tender. Women shouldn't brush their breasts.

- Start gently

- Always brush towards your heart

- Start with the soles of your feet and up each leg

- Brush from the hands along your arms to your shoulders

- Brush upwards on the buttocks and lower back

- Use a gentle motion on the tummy towards the centre

- Brush from the back of the neck to the front and gently on the chest towards the heart

Note: if you have any medical condition, then check with your doctor before trying skin brushing.

Epsom salt baths

Epsom salt is named after a saline spring at Epsom in Surrey, England and is a naturally occurring mineral compound of magnesium and sulfate. Studies have shown that these minerals are readily absorbed through the skin and also may help with the elimination of toxins.

An Epsom salt bath a couple of times a week brings many benefits:

- Helps with inflammation
- Eases stress and relaxes the body
- Relieves aches and pains
- Improves the body's absorption of nutrients
- May help with constipation

Aromatherapy massage

A full-body aromatherapy massage or session of reflexology can do wonders for your digestion. And treating yourself to a natural essential oils body oil to use after the bath at home is the perfect way to pamper yourself through the cleanse (or at any time!). A ginger-based oil is particularly good for warming tired muscles, rose is excellent for soothing emotions and lavender will help send you off into blissful sleep.

Self-care rituals

Throughout the day, add a few small but significant rituals, such as switching off from technology for a few minutes while you sit quietly with a cup of tea. Aim to get outside and go for a walk every day; no matter how short the walk, being in the fresh air is a tonic. Even juicing itself feels like a ritual or a meditation – all you need to do in the moment is juice your vegetables, nothing else! When you simplify your diet for a few days, you might find that you are more aware than usual of your senses – you can make the most of this by breathing in the scents of a garden, or using a pulse point essential oil, listening to the birds sing in the morning, savouring flavours, and giving yourself a relaxing foot massage.

How to deal with cravings

It doesn't take the body long to get over cravings for things like sugar and caffeine, but the initial hit of a craving can be hard to ignore. It's a really good idea to gradually wean yourself off tea and coffee and refined sugars in the few days before going on a juice cleanse. If you experience cravings during the cleanse, there is an excellent visualization technique that can help:

- When you experience a feeling of craving, find a quiet place for a couple of minutes.

- Take three gentle, deep breaths and relax your shoulders.

- Now use the powers of your imagination and describe to yourself how it will feel to complete today on the juice cleanse (this can also work for any lifestyle change).

- Imagine how a sense of renewed energy feels and what it allows you to do.

- Imagine a feeling of clear-headedness and a lightness in your digestion.

- If this brings a smile to your face, go ahead and smile.

By distracting your mind and your senses away from the craving to positive thoughts and feelings about the healthy change you're making, the cravings loosen their hold and gradually will drift away. The key is to focus on all the enjoyable parts of making a change.

What if you get headaches?

By weaning yourself off caffeine and sugar before you start the cleanse, you will be less likely to experience headaches. The nuts and nut milk included in this cleanse also help by adding good fats and protein. If you do experience headaches, try these natural solutions:

- Epsom salt bath
- Drink plenty of water
- Move your body with gentle walks, stretching and yoga
- Allow yourself plenty of rest

- Add some ground flaxseeds or flaxseed oil to your juices

CHAPTER 5

7-DAY JUICE AND SOUP CLEANSE

This chapter outlines the second phase of the 10-day cleanse, where for the remaining 7 days soups can be added. The soup cleanse can also be implemented separately to the juice cleanse, if the thought of only consuming juice and a few nuts feels too much! Inspired by starting the day with celery juice, the ingredients included in this cleanse are a combination of anti-inflammatory, gut-friendly and bloat-busting. This plan is also vegetarian and gluten-free and the only dairy is in kefir and yoghurt, which are considered to be easy on the digestion (but do omit if you are vegan or intolerant to all dairy - and replace with coconut kefir and vegan yoghurt). Eating this way for a couple of days each week is also an excellent way to allow your body to come back into balance and it encourages you to give your kitchen a good cleanse at the same time.

SEVEN-DAY MENU

Day one

Warm water and lemon juice

Celery Juice, see page 48

Bircher Muesli (make enough for 2 servings, so that you can have some the next day), see page 76

Zinger Juice, see page 49

Miso Soup, see page 84

Beetroot and Caraway Soup, (make enough for 2 servings), see page 82

Day two

Warm water and lemon juice

Celery Juice, see page 48

Bircher Muesli, see page 76

Green Juice, see page 50

Beetroot and Caraway Soup, see page 82

Kitchari (make enough for 3 servings), see page 89

Day three

Warm water and lemon juice

Celery Juice, see page 48

Green Smoothie Bowl, see page 72

Miso Mushroom Soup (make enough for 2 servings), see page 85

Zinger Juice, see page 49

Kitchari, see page 89

Day four

Warm water and lemon juice

Celery Juice, see page 48

Spiced Eggs with Spinach and Avocado, see page 78

Green Juice, see page 50

Kitchari, see page 89

Fast evening*, see page 67

Day five

Warm water and lemon juice

Celery Juice, see page 48

Berry Kefir, see page 75

Miso Mushroom Soup, see page 85

Ginger, Turmeric and Carrot Soup
(make enough for 2 servings), see page 87

Day six

Warm water and lemon juice

Celery Juice, see page 48

Digestive Smoothie, see page 74

Ginger, Turmeric and Carrot Soup, see page 87

Nut Milk, see page 53

Aduki Bean Masala (make enough for 2
servings), see page 92

Day seven

Warm water and lemon juice

Celery Juice, see page 48

Spiced Eggs with Spinach and Avocado,
see page 78

Sunshine Juice, see page 50

Miso Soup, see page 84

Aduki Bean Masala, see page 92

*Fast evening

One evening of fasting is included during this
plan as it's not something that is easy to get
used to very quickly, but when your willpower
is at its height it's the perfect time to try it. Our
modern lifestyles often encourage us to run out
of the door in the morning without breakfast,
eat very little during the day and try to catch up
in the evening. For our bodies, the more often
we can do the opposite and take the time for a
good breakfast, a decent lunch and then a light,
early supper, the better we will feel. Ideally, we
would eat our complex carbs earlier in the day

and go for protein and veg in the evening, as we need energy during the day and then can lighten things up for our digestion overnight.

Teas
Fennel

Nettle

Dandelion

Green

Fresh mint

Infused waters
Cucumber

Rosemary

Mint

Lime

Kombucha is a fermented drink made with beneficial bacteria, so is a good gut-friendly choice.

For a warm health-boosting drink add a little turmeric root, lemon juice and fresh root ginger to hot water.

THE RECIPES

BREAKFASTS

Green smoothie bowl

This smoothie bowl is packed with fruit and vegetables, with the added optional extra of a spoonful of matcha, which is a fine powder made from young green tea leaves. The word 'matcha' translates as 'powdered tea'. All green tea is high in antioxidants, and matcha tea has been shown to be the highest food-level source of catechins, a group of anti-inflammatory antioxidants that help prevent heart disease. Catechins also counteract the effects of free radicals from the environment, such as pollution and the sun's damaging UV rays.

SERVES I

½ avocado, stoned and peeled
½ banana, sliced and frozen
¼ cucumber, roughly chopped
25g (1oz) baby spinach leaves
Approximately 50ml (2fl oz) coconut water
1 teaspoon matcha powder
Squeeze of lime juice

To serve
Live natural yoghurt
Chopped hazelnuts

Place all the smoothie ingredients in a blender
and blend until thick and smooth. Add
enough coconut water to achieve your desired
consistency. Serve topped with the yoghurt and
chopped hazelnuts.

Digestive smoothie

Pineapple, celery and cucumber are all excellent for digestion, while flaxseeds are a good plant-based source of omega-3 essential fatty acids.

SERVES 1

100g (3½oz) fresh pineapple, peeled and chopped
2 celery sticks, chopped
2 tablespoons lime juice
1 tablespoon flaxseeds, soaked overnight
Ice cubes or water (optional)

Put all the ingredients into a blender and blend until completely smooth. Add ice cubes or a little water, if desired.

Berry kefir

Bananas are are prebiotic and so have been shown to help increase healthy gut bacteria. And kefir is a type of cultured yoghurt that contains high levels of healthy bacteria. You can also add spinach leaves to this smoothie for an extra green punch – you won't taste the difference.

SERVES 1

100g (3½oz) frozen blueberries
100ml (3½fl oz) kefir
1 tablespoon almond butter
½ banana, peeled
A little water

Put all the ingredients, except the water into a blender and blend together until smooth, adding a little water until you reach the desired smoothie consistency.

Bircher muesli

Bircher Muesli takes its name from Dr Maximilian Bircher-Brenner, a Swiss physician and pioneer in nutritional research around 1900. Dr Bircher-Brenner set up a sanatorium called Vital Force, based on the German lifestyle-reform movement which is based on living in harmony with nature. Instead of the usual diet of much meat and potatoes, he recommended fruit, vegetables and nuts.

You can make double the quantity of soaked oats and store the extra portion, covered, in the fridge for another morning. Just stir in the apple, lime juice and yoghurt as needed later. Add fresh berries if you fancy.

SERVES 2

100g (3½oz) gluten-free oats
1 tablespoon flaxseeds
1 tablespoon chia seeds
¼ teaspoon ground cinnamon
100ml (3½fl oz) unsweetened almond milk
200ml (7fl oz) water
Few drops of vanilla extract
1 apple, grated
juice of ½ lime
2 tablespoons natural yoghurt
1 tablespoon hazelnuts, roughly chopped

The night before, mix together the oats, seeds, cinnamon, almond milk, water and vanilla extract in a large bowl, cover and chill in the refrigerator overnight.

In the morning, grate the apple and stir into the soaked oats, along with the lime juice, yoghurt and chopped hazelnuts.

Spiced eggs with spinach and avocado

Spices are excellent for perking up your digestive fire.

SERVES I

2 eggs

¼ teaspoon ground turmeric

I small or ½ large ripe avocado

Squeeze of lemon juice

2 teaspoons coconut oil (or olive oil)

40g (1½oz) baby spinach leaves (or kale)

Sea salt and freshly ground black pepper

Crack the eggs into a bowl and whisk with the turmeric and a good pinch of black pepper.

Cut the avocado in half and remove the stone. Spoon out the flesh and mash with lemon juice and a little salt.

Melt half the coconut oil in a small non-stick frying pan and half in a large frying pan. Add the eggs into the small pan and add a pinch of salt. Leave for a few seconds for the eggs to start cooking on the bottom and gently fold over with a spatula. Remove the eggs from the heat while just undercooked as they will continue to cook in the residual heat.

Meanwhile, sauté the spinach leaves in the large pan for just a minute to wilt.

Serve the eggs on top of the wilted spinach, with the mashed avocado on the side.

THE RECIPES

SOUPS

Beetroot and caraway soup

Beetroot is considered a tonifying food by traditional medicines including Traditional Chinese Medicine, and caraway seeds are good for digestion, too.

SERVES 2

500g (1lb 2 oz) beetroot, washed

1 tablespoon apple cider vinegar

1 tablespoon olive oil

1 tablespoon caraway seeds

1 leek, top and tailed and sliced

300ml (10fl oz) hot water or vegetable stock

2 tablespoons lemon juice

Sea salt flakes and freshly ground black pepper

Preheat the oven to 200°C (350°F, Gas Mark 4.

Place the beetroot in a roasting tray and add
2.5cm (1in) of water in the bottom of the
tray. Sprinkle over the apple cider vinegar
and some salt and cover with foil. Roast for
approximately 90 minutes, until the beetroot
can be easily pierced with a knife.

Remove from the oven, allow the beetroot to
cool, then rub off the skins and chop roughly.

Heat the olive oil in a pan and add the caraway
seeds. When the seeds start to pop, add the leek,
sautéing until soft, about 10 minutes.

Add the roasted beetroot, measured hot water
or stock, and season with black pepper and salt.
Simmer for 15 minutes, allow to cool a little and
then transfer to a blender and blend until smooth.

Add the lemon juice and serve.

Miso soup

Miso soup is very versatile as you can make the base with a miso paste and then add any of the following ingredients that you fancy.

1 teaspoon miso paste
Baby spinach leaves
Firm tofu, cut into cubes
Edamame beans, blanched
Kimchi
Cooked shiitake mushrooms
Seaweed strips
Cooked brown rice

To make the base, add a heaped teaspoon of miso paste to a measuring jug. Boil a kettle of water and add just a little to the miso paste and stir in to make a looser paste. Add 250ml just-boiled water to make your miso soup base.

Miso mushroom soup

Miso paste is a type of fermented soy bean and is considered very good for your digestion.

SERVES 2

2 tablespoons olive oil
50g (1¾oz) shiitake mushrooms
200g (7oz) chestnut mushrooms
1 teaspoon apple cider vinegar
300ml (10fl oz) hot vegetable stock
10g (¼ oz) white miso paste
160ml (5fl oz) almond milk
1 teaspoon fresh rosemary, chopped

Heat the oil in a large saucepan over a low-medium heat. Add all the mushrooms and cook for 10 minutes.

Deglaze the pan with the apple cider vinegar, remove about a quarter of the mushrooms and set aside. Add the hot stock and the miso paste

to the pan, stir through and continue to cook for
another 5 minutes.

Remove from the heat and set aside for 10
minutes. Add the almond milk and blend
until smooth.

To serve, gently reheat the soup and the reserved
mushrooms, separately, adding a little chopped
fresh rosemary to the mushrooms while
warming through. Divide between bowls
and serve.

Ginger, turmeric and carrot soup

This carrot soup is very warming and so is easy on the digestion. It is good to include a rainbow of colours in your diet as much as possible, so not all green! If you buy organic carrots, you can simply wash and rub the skins; if the carrots are not organic then peel them.

SERVES 2

1 tablespoon olive oil

½ onion, chopped

1 celery stick, chopped

1 teaspoon peeled and grated fresh root ginger

1 teaspoon ground turmeric (or grated fresh root turmeric)

250g (9oz) carrots, roughly chopped

400ml (14fl oz) hot vegetable stock

40g(1½oz) almond or hazelnuts, roughly chopped

½ teaspoon mild chilli powder (optional)

Sea salt flakes and freshly ground black pepper

Heat the oil in a saucepan over a low-medium heat, add the onion and celery and sauté for about 10 minutes until soft. Add the ginger, turmeric and a good pinch of black pepper and stir through before adding the carrots.

Continue to stir the carrots for another couple of minutes and then add the stock. Bring to the boil, reduce the heat and simmer for 10–15 minutes, or until the carrots are tender.

Allow to cool a little, before transferring to a blender and process until smooth. Taste and adjust the seasoning.

Mix the chopped nuts with the mild chilli powder (if using) and dry roast in a frying pan for a couple of minutes over a low heat.

Serve the soup in bowls, scattered with the spiced nuts.

Kitchari

This recipe is based on an Ayurvedic cleansing soup, kitchari. It is made with soaked mung beans, which are becoming more readily available in supermarkets and are easily found in Asian supermarkets and health-food stores. Mung beans are thought to be particularly good for alleviating excess water retention. It is a type of dhal and can also be made in a big batch for quick, healthy meals to enjoy during the week.

SERVES 3

200g (7oz) green mung beans, rinsed and soaked overnight

1 teaspoon ground turmeric

¼ teaspoon ground black pepper

¼ teaspoon asafoetida

Zest and juice of 1 lemon

20g (1oz) coconut oil (or butter)

1 onion, sliced

¼ teaspoon mustard seeds

¼ teaspoon cumin seeds

¼ teaspoon fennel seeds

¼ teaspoon nigella seeds

6 dried curry leaves

Sea salt flakes

To serve

Natural yoghurt

Baby spinach leaves

Rinse and drain the mung beans and put into a large saucepan with 1 litre (1¾ pints) of water.

Add the turmeric, black pepper, a good pinch of salt and the asafoetida and bring to the boil. Reduce to a low simmer and cook for about an hour, or until the beans are soft. Add the lemon juice and zest, half the coconut oil or butter and take off the heat.

Heat the remaining oil or butter in a frying pan and cook the onions for a few minutes before adding all the spices and cooking for a couple more minutes until all the aromas of the spices have been released.

Add the spiced onions to the kitchari and give it a single stir (rather than fully combining the ingredients).

To serve, ladle into bowls and top with a spoonful of natural yoghurt and some baby spinach leaves.

Aduki bean masala

Aduki beans are diuretic and so this recipe is
excellent for banishing the bloat.

SERVES 2

1 tablespoon olive oil

1 large or 2 medium leeks, top, tailed and sliced

1 head of fennel, sliced

Good pinch of sea salt flakes

½ teaspoon cumin seeds

½ teaspoon fennel seeds

½ teaspoon mustard seeds

½ teaspoon mild chilli powder

400g (14oz) can aduki beans, rinsed and drained

200g (7oz) passata

Natural yoghurt, to serve

Heat the oil in a large, heavy-bottomed saucepan. Add the leeks and fennel and sauté on a low heat for about 10 minutes with the lid on, removing it to stir every couple of minutes.

Add the salt and spices and stir for a couple of minutes while the aromas are released.

Add the beans to the pan along with the passata. Stir through everything gently, bring to a simmer and cook for about 30 minutes or until the vegetables are tender.

Allow to rest, covered, for a few minutes before ladling into bowls and serving topped with a spoonful of natural yoghurt.

GOOD LUCK!

I wish you all the best of luck on your health journey and hope the lessons learned from this book serve you well. Get juicing!

References

7 'It's current spell in the spotlight is largely down to':

medicalmedium.com

18 'A further rat study':

https://www.ncbi.nlm.nih.gov/pmc/articles/PMC3684138/

19 'Other studies on rats fed a high fat diet':

https://www.ncbi.nlm.nih.gov/pmc/articles/PMC3684138/

19 'Other studies on rats fed a high fat diet have demonstrated':

http://go.galegroup.com/ps/anonymous?id=GALE%-
7CA392176383&sid=googleScholar&v=2.1&it=r&link-
access=fulltext&issn=19950756&p=AONE&sw=w&auth-
Count=1&isAnonymousEntry=true

19 'Celery is high in antioxidant flavones and polyphenols':

https://www.ncbi.nlm.nih.gov/pubmed/28423952

19 'A study published in Molecular Nutrition & Food Research':

https://onlinelibrary.wiley.com/doi/full/10.1002/mnfr.201400705

20 'The apigenin in celery is also thought to stimulate neurogenesis':

https://www.tandfonline.com/doi/abs/10.1517/135437709

027212 79?journalCode=ietp20

20 'Liver enzymes help break down proteins for the body':

https://www.ncbi.nlm.nih.gov/pmc/articles/PMC3113355/

22 'Certain chemical constituents may':

https://www.ncbi.nlm.nih.gov/pubmed/20645778

22 'inflammation and increases cancer risk':

https://www.ncbi.nlm.nih.gov/pubmed/24374236

22 'A study in Current Cancer Drug Targets':

https://www.ncbi.nlm.nih.gov/pubmed/18991571

22 'A 2009 study on rats found':

https://www.ncbi.nlm.nih.gov/pmc/articles/PMC6254272/

INDEX